WHOLESOME MEDITERRANEAN DELIGHTS:

30 INSPIRING RECIPES FOR A BALANCED LIFESTYLE AND LONGEVITY

WILLIAMS .C. HARDWICK

TABLE OF CONTENT

INTRODUCTION

In the sun-kissed lands of the Mediterranean, where olive groves dance in the breeze and azure seas beckon with tranquility, a culinary journey unfolds. "Wholesome Mediterranean Delights: 30 Inspiring Recipes for a Balanced Lifestyle and Longevity" invites you to savor the essence of a region renowned for its flavorful tapestry and healthful traditions.Embark on a voyage through the vibrant markets and quaint villages, where generations have embraced a lifestyle harmonized by the art of mindful eating. In this culinary odyssey, we unearth 30 handcrafted recipes that not only tantalize the taste buds but also nurture the body and soul. Each dish is a celebration of the bountiful gifts bestowed by the Mediterranean, combining fresh herbs, ripe produce, and heart-healthy olive oil in perfect harmony.From the sun-drenched coasts of Greece to the rustic charm of Italian kitchens, these recipes encapsulate the secrets to a balanced life, promoting well-being and longevity. Discover the joy of preparing and savoring dishes that honor the time-tested principles of the Mediterranean diet, fostering a connection between food, community, and the simple pleasures of life.

As you turn the pages of "Wholesome Mediterranean Delights," let the aroma of basil, the zest of citrus, and the warmth of spices transport you to a realm where culinary craftsmanship meets a commitment to wellness. Embrace the Mediterranean spirit, and embark on a delightful journey toward a healthier, more wholesome lifestyle.

30 INSPIRING RECIPES FOR A BALANCED LIFESTYLE AND LONGEVITY

1. Mediterranean Chickpea Salad:

INGREDIENTS:

- Chickpeas
- Cucumber
- Cherry tomatoes
- Red onion
- Feta cheese
- Kalamata olives
- Olive oil
- Lemon juice
- Oregano

INSTRUCTIONS:

1.   Rinse and drain canned chickpeas.

2.   Dice cucumber, halve cherry tomatoes, finely chop red onion, and crumble feta cheese.

3.   Combine chickpeas, cucumber, cherry tomatoes, red onion, feta cheese, and Kalamata olives in a large bowl.

4.   In a small bowl, whisk together olive oil, lemon juice, and oregano.

5.   Drizzle the dressing over the salad and toss gently to combine.

6.   Serve chilled.

2. Greek Quinoa Bowl:

INGREDIENTS:

- Quinoa
- Spinach
- Cherry tomatoes
- Cucumber
- Red onion
- Feta cheese
- Kalamata olives
- Olive oil
- Lemon

INSTRUCTIONS:

1.   Cook quinoa according to package instructions and let it cool.

2.   In a large bowl, combine cooked quinoa, fresh spinach, halved cherry tomatoes, diced cucumber, sliced red onion, crumbled feta cheese, and Kalamata olives.

3.   In a small bowl, whisk together olive oil and the juice of one lemon.

4.   Drizzle the dressing over the quinoa mixture and toss gently to coat.

5.   Serve as a refreshing and nutritious bowl.

3. Mediterranean Grilled Chicken:

INGREDIENTS:

- Chicken breasts
- Garlic
- Lemon
- Olive oil
- Oregano
- Rosemary
- Salt and pepper

INSTRUCTIONS:

1.   In a bowl, combine minced garlic, the juice of one lemon, olive oil, dried oregano, rosemary, salt, and pepper to create a marinade.

2.   Place chicken breasts in a shallow dish and coat with the marinade. Allow it to marinate for at least 30 minutes.

3.   Preheat the grill to medium-high heat.

4.   Grill the chicken breasts for about 6-8 minutes per side or until fully cooked.

5.   Let the chicken rest for a few minutes before serving.

4. Caprese Salad:
INGREDIENTS:

- Tomatoes
- Fresh mozzarella
- Fresh basil
- Balsamic glaze
- Olive oil
- Salt and pepper

INSTRUCTIONS:

1. Slice tomatoes and fresh mozzarella into even thickness.

2. Arrange tomato and mozzarella slices on a serving platter, alternating and slightly overlapping.

3. Tuck fresh basil leaves between the tomato and mozzarella slices.

4. Drizzle with balsamic glaze and olive oil.

5. Season with salt and pepper to taste.

6. Serve immediately as a light and flavorful salad.

5. Mediterranean Eggplant Dip (Baba Ganoush)

INGREDIENTS:

- Eggplant
- Tahini
- Garlic
- Lemon juice
- Olive oil
- Salt and cumin

INSTRUCTIONS:

1.   Preheat the oven to 400°F (200°C).

2.   Pierce the eggplant several times with a fork and place it on a baking sheet.

3.   Roast the eggplant in the oven for about 45-50 minutes or until the skin is charred and the flesh is soft.

4.   Let the eggplant cool, then peel off the skin and mash the flesh.

5.   In a bowl, combine the mashed eggplant, tahini, minced garlic, lemon juice, olive oil, salt, and a pinch of cumin.

6.   Mix well and refrigerate before serving.

6. Mediterranean Baked Cod:

- **INGREDIENTS:**
    - Cod fillets
    - Cherry tomatoes
    - Kalamata olives
    - Red onion
    - Garlic
    - Olive oil
    - Lemon
    - Oregano

INSTRUCTIONS:

1. Preheat the oven to 375°F (190°C).

2. Place cod fillets in a baking dish.

3. Surround the cod with halved cherry tomatoes, sliced Kalamata olives, diced red onion, and minced garlic.

4. Drizzle with olive oil and lemon juice. Sprinkle with oregano.

5. Bake for 20-25 minutes or until the cod is cooked through and flakes easily.

6. Serve with a side of quinoa or couscous.

INGREDIENTS:

- Lentils
- Carrots
- Celery
- Onion
- Garlic
- Tomatoes
- Vegetable broth
- Cumin
- Coriander
- Olive oil

INSTRUCTIONS:

1.   In a large pot, sauté diced onions and minced garlic in olive oil until softened.

2.   Add chopped carrots, celery, and diced tomatoes to the pot. Cook for a few minutes.

3.   Rinse lentils and add them to the pot along with vegetable broth, cumin, and coriander.

4.   Bring to a boil, then reduce heat and simmer for 25-30 minutes or until lentils are tender.

5.   Season with salt and pepper to taste.

6.   Serve hot, optionally garnished with fresh parsley.

8. Spinach and Feta Stuffed Chicken Breast:

INGREDIENTS:

- Chicken breasts
- Spinach
- Feta cheese
- Garlic
- Olive oil
- Lemon juice
- Oregano
- Salt and pepper

INSTRUCTIONS*:*

1.   Preheat the oven to 375°F (190°C).

2.   Butterfly chicken breasts by making a horizontal cut through the thickest part.

3.   In a skillet, sauté minced garlic in olive oil until fragrant.

4.   Add fresh spinach and cook until wilted.

5.   Remove from heat and stir in crumbled feta.

6.   Stuff each chicken breast with the spinach and feta mixture.

7.   Place the stuffed chicken breasts in a baking dish.

8.   Drizzle with lemon juice, sprinkle with oregano, salt, and pepper.

9.   Bake for 25-30 minutes or until chicken is fully cooked.

10.   Allow the chicken to rest before slicing and serving.

9. Mediterranean Chickpea and Vegetable Skewers:

INGREDIENTS:

- Chickpeas (canned, drained)
- Cherry tomatoes
- Bell peppers (assorted colors)
- Red onion
- Zucchini
- Olive oil
- Lemon juice
- Oregano
- Salt and pepper

INSTRUCTIONS:

1.   Preheat the grill or grill pan.

2.   Thread canned chickpeas and assorted vegetables onto skewers, alternating.

3.   In a small bowl, whisk together olive oil, lemon juice, oregano, salt, and pepper.

4.   Brush the skewers with the olive oil mixture.

5.   Grill the skewers for 10-12 minutes, turning occasionally, until vegetables are tender.

6.   Serve the skewers with a side of tzatziki sauce.

10. Greek Tzatziki Sauce:

INGREDIENTS:

- Greek yogurt
- Cucumber
- Garlic
- Lemon juice
- Fresh dill
- Olive oil
- Salt and pepper

INSTRUCTIONS:

1.	Grate cucumber and squeeze out excess liquid using a clean kitchen towel.

2.	In a bowl, combine Greek yogurt, grated cucumber, minced garlic, lemon juice, chopped fresh dill, olive oil, salt, and pepper.

3.	Mix well until all ingredients are evenly incorporated.

4.	Refrigerate for at least 30 minutes before serving.

5.	Stir before serving, and adjust salt and pepper to taste.

11. Mediterranean Shrimp Pasta:
INGREDIENTS:

- Shrimp
- Whole wheat pasta
- Cherry tomatoes
- Spinach
- Garlic
- Olive oil
- Lemon zest
- Red pepper flakes

INSTRUCTIONS:

1.   Cook whole wheat pasta according to package instructions.

2.   In a large skillet, sauté shrimp and minced garlic in olive oil until shrimp are pink and cooked through.

3.   Add halved cherry tomatoes and fresh spinach to the skillet. Cook until spinach wilts.

4.   Toss the cooked pasta into the skillet with the shrimp, tomatoes, and spinach.

5.   Drizzle with olive oil and sprinkle with lemon zest and red pepper flakes.

6.   Toss everything together until well combined.

7.   Serve warm with an additional sprinkle of red pepper flakes if desired.

12.   Mediterranean   Roasted Vegetables:

INGREDIENTS:

- Eggplant
- Zucchini
- Cherry tomatoes
- Red onion
- Bell peppers (assorted colors)
- Garlic
- Olive oil
- Balsamic vinegar

INSTRUCTIONS:

1.   Preheat the oven to 425°F (220°C).

2.   Cut eggplant, zucchini, cherry tomatoes, red onion, and bell peppers into bite-sized pieces.

3.   Place the vegetables on a baking sheet, ensuring they are spread evenly.

4.   Drizzle with olive oil and balsamic vinegar. Toss to coat.

5.   Roast in the oven for 25-30 minutes or until the vegetables are tender and slightly caramelized.

6.   Remove from the oven and let cool slightly before serving.

13. Mediterranean Hummus Wrap:

INGREDIENTS:

- Whole wheat wrap
- Hummus
- Cherry tomatoes
- Cucumber
- Red bell pepper
- Red onion
- Kalamata olives
- Feta cheese
- Olive oil
- Fresh parsley

INSTRUCTIONS:

1.   Spread a generous layer of hummus on a whole wheat wrap.

2.   Layer sliced cherry tomatoes, cucumber, red bell pepper, red onion, Kalamata olives, and crumbled feta cheese.

3.   Drizzle with olive oil and sprinkle with fresh parsley.

4.   Fold the sides of the wrap and roll it tightly.

5.   Slice in half diagonally and enjoy this delicious and portable Mediterranean meal.

14. Mediterranean Stuffed Peppers:
INGREDIENTS:

- Bell peppers
- Quinoa
- Chickpeas
- Cherry tomatoes
- Red onion
- Feta cheese
- Kalamata olives
- Olive oil
- Lemon juice
- Oregano
- Salt and pepper

INSTRUCTIONS:

1.   Preheat the oven to 375°F (190°C).

2.   Cut bell peppers in half lengthwise and remove seeds.

3.   In a bowl, mix cooked quinoa, chickpeas, halved cherry tomatoes, diced red onion, crumbled feta cheese, and sliced Kalamata olives.

4.   In a small bowl, whisk together olive oil, lemon juice, oregano, salt, and pepper.

5.   Stuff each bell pepper half with the quinoa mixture.

6.   Drizzle the stuffed peppers with the olive oil mixture.

7.   Bake for 25-30 minutes or until the peppers are tender=

15. Mediterranean Zucchini Noodles with Pesto:

INGREDIENTS:

- Zucchini
- Cherry tomatoes
- Pine nuts
- Pesto sauce
- Parmesan cheese
- Olive oil
- Lemon zest
- Salt and pepper

INSTRUCTIONS:

1. Spiralize zucchini into noodles.

2. In a skillet, sauté zucchini noodles with halved cherry tomatoes in olive oil until just tender.

3. Stir in pesto sauce and pine nuts.

4. Cook for an additional 2-3 minutes.

5. Sprinkle with freshly grated Parmesan, lemon zest, salt, and pepper.

6. Toss well before serving for a light and flavorful dish.

16. Mediterranean Chickpea Patties:

INGREDIENTS:

- Chickpeas (canned, drained)
- Red onion
- Garlic
- Fresh parsley
- Cumin
- Coriander
- Whole wheat breadcrumbs
- Olive oil
- Greek yogurt (for serving)

INSTRUCTIONS:

1.   In a food processor, blend chickpeas, chopped red onion, minced garlic, fresh parsley, cumin, coriander, and whole wheat breadcrumbs until well combined.

2.   Form the mixture into patties.

3.   Heat olive oil in a skillet over medium heat.

4.   Cook chickpea patties for 3-4 minutes on each side or until golden brown.

5.   Serve with a dollop of Greek yogurt.

17. Mediterranean Orzo Salad:
INGREDIENTS:

- Orzo pasta
- Cherry tomatoes
- Cucumber
- Red onion
- Kalamata olives
- Feta cheese
- Olive oil
- Lemon juice
- Oregano
- Salt and pepper

INSTRUCTIONS:

1.   Cook orzo pasta according to package instructions. Let it cool.

2.   Dice cherry tomatoes, cucumber, and red onion.

3.   In a large bowl, combine cooked orzo, diced vegetables, sliced Kalamata olives, and crumbled feta cheese.

4.   In a small bowl, whisk together olive oil, lemon juice, oregano, salt, and pepper.

5.   Drizzle the dressing over the orzo salad and toss gently to combine.

18. Mediterranean Roasted Red Pepper Dip:

INGREDIENTS:

- Roasted red peppers (jarred)
- Cannellini beans (canned, drained)
- Garlic
- Lemon juice
- Tahini
- Olive oil
- Cumin
- Paprika
- Salt and pepper

INSTRUCTIONS:

1. In a food processor, combine roasted red peppers, cannellini beans, minced garlic, lemon juice, tahini, olive oil, cumin, paprika, salt, and pepper.

2. Blend until smooth and creamy.

3. Adjust seasoning to taste.

4. Serve as a dip with pita bread or vegetable sticks.

19. Mediterranean Baked Falafel:

INGREDIENTS:

- Chickpeas (canned, drained)
- Red onion
- Garlic
- Fresh parsley
- Cumin
- Coriander
- Baking powder
- Olive oil
- Greek yogurt (for serving)

INSTRUCTIONS:

1. Preheat the oven to 375°F (190°C).

2. In a food processor, blend chickpeas, chopped red onion, minced garlic, fresh parsley, cumin, coriander, and baking powder until a coarse mixture forms.

3. Form the mixture into small patties and place on a baking sheet.

4. Brush the falafel patties with olive oil.

5. Bake for 20-25 minutes or until golden brown.

6. Serve with a side of Greek yogurt.

20. Mediterranean Couscous Salad:

INGREDIENTS:

- Couscous
- Cherry tomatoes
- Cucumber
- Red bell pepper
- Red onion
- Feta cheese
- Kalamata olives
- Olive oil
- Lemon juice
- Fresh mint
- Salt and pepper

INSTRUCTIONS:

1. Cook couscous according to package instructions. Let it cool.

2. Dice cherry tomatoes, cucumber, red bell pepper, and red onion.

3. In a large bowl, combine cooked couscous, diced vegetables, crumbled feta cheese, sliced Kalamata olives, and fresh mint.

4. In a small bowl, whisk together olive oil and lemon juice.

5. Drizzle the dressing over the couscous salad and toss gently to combine.

6. Season with salt and pepper to taste.

21. Mediterranean Shrimp and Vegetable Skewers:

INGREDIENTS:

- Shrimp
- Cherry tomatoes
- Bell peppers (assorted colors)
- Red onion
- Zucchini
- Olive oil
- Lemon juice
- Garlic
- Oregano
- Salt and pepper

INSTRUCTIONS:

1.   Preheat the grill or grill pan.

2.   Thread shrimp and assorted vegetables onto skewers.

3.   In a small bowl, whisk together olive oil, lemon juice, minced garlic, oregano, salt, and pepper.

4.   Brush the skewers with the olive oil mixture.

5.   Grill for 5-7 minutes, turning occasionally, until the shrimp are opaque and the vegetables are tender.

6.   Serve over a bed of quinoa or couscous.

## 22.	**Mediterranean	Stuffed Artichokes:**

- *Ingredients:*
    - Artichokes
    - Quinoa
    - Chickpeas
    - Sun-dried tomatoes
    - Feta cheese
    - Fresh basil
    - Lemon
    - Olive oil
    - Garlic
    - Salt and pepper

INSTRUCTIONS:

1.   Preheat the oven to 375°F (190°C).

2.   Prepare artichokes by trimming the tops and removing the outer tough leaves.

3.   In a bowl, mix cooked quinoa, chickpeas, chopped sun-dried tomatoes, crumbled feta cheese, chopped fresh basil, lemon zest, and a drizzle of olive oil.

4.   Stuff the artichokes with the quinoa mixture.

5.   Place the stuffed artichokes in a baking dish, add a splash of water, cover with foil, and bake for 45-50 minutes or until the artichokes are tender.

23. Mediterranean Tuna Salad:
INGREDIENTS:

- Canned tuna
- Cherry tomatoes
- Cucumber
- Red onion
- Kalamata olives
- Feta cheese
- Olive oil
- Lemon juice
- Oregano
- Salt and pepper

INSTRUCTIONS:

1.   Drain the canned tuna and place it in a large bowl.

2.   Dice cherry tomatoes, cucumber, red onion, and slice Kalamata olives.

3.   Add the diced vegetables to the tuna along with crumbled feta cheese.

4.   In a small bowl, whisk together olive oil, lemon juice, oregano, salt, and pepper.

5.   Pour the dressing over the tuna mixture and toss gently to combine.

6.   Serve over a bed of mixed greens for a refreshing tuna salad.

24. *Mediterranean Lemon Herb Chicken Skewers:*

INGREDIENTS:

- Chicken breasts, cut into cubes
- Cherry tomatoes
- Red onion
- Bell peppers (assorted colors)
- Lemon
- Olive oil
- Garlic
- Fresh herbs (rosemary, thyme, oregano)
- Salt and pepper

INSTRUCTIONS:

1.   In a bowl, combine cubed chicken, halved cherry tomatoes, sliced red onion, and diced bell peppers.

2.   In a separate bowl, whisk together olive oil, lemon juice, minced garlic, chopped fresh herbs, salt, and pepper.

3.   Marinate the chicken and vegetables in the lemon herb mixture for at least 30 minutes.

4.   Thread the marinated chicken and vegetables onto skewers.

5.   Grill for 10-12 minutes, turning occasionally, until the chicken is cooked through and has a nice char.

6.   Serve with a side of quinoa or couscous.

25. Mediterranean Artichoke and Spinach Dip:

INGREDIENTS:

- Frozen chopped spinach, thawed and drained
- Artichoke hearts, chopped
- Cream cheese
- Greek yogurt
- Feta cheese
- Garlic
- Olive oil
- Lemon juice
- Salt and pepper

INSTRUCTIONS:

1.   Preheat the oven to 375°F (190°C).

2.   In a mixing bowl, combine thawed and drained chopped spinach, chopped artichoke hearts, softened cream cheese, Greek yogurt, crumbled feta cheese, minced garlic, olive oil, and lemon juice.

3.   Mix until all ingredients are well combined.

4.   Transfer the mixture to a baking dish and bake for 25-30 minutes or until the dip is hot and bubbly.

5.   Serve with pita chips or vegetable sticks.

26. Mediterranean Pita Pocket with Falafel:

INGREDIENTS:

- Whole wheat pita pockets
- Baked falafel
- Cherry tomatoes
- Cucumber
- Red onion
- Greek yogurt
- Fresh mint
- Lemon juice
- Olive oil
- Salt and pepper

INSTRUCTIONS:

11.   Cut the top off each pita pocket to create an opening.

12.   Fill each pita with baked falafel, sliced cherry tomatoes, diced cucumber, and thinly sliced red onion.

13.   In a small bowl, mix Greek yogurt with chopped fresh mint, lemon juice, olive oil, salt, and pepper.

14.   Drizzle the yogurt sauce into each pita pocket.

15.   Serve immediately for a satisfying and flavorful handheld meal.

27. Mediterranean Herb and Lemon Quinoa:

INGREDIENTS:

- Quinoa
- Cherry tomatoes
- Cucumber
- Red bell pepper
- Red onion
- Feta cheese
- Olive oil
- Lemon juice
- Fresh parsley
- Salt and pepper

INSTRUCTIONS:

11.   Cook quinoa according to package instructions. Let it cool.

12.   Dice cherry tomatoes, cucumber, red bell pepper, and red onion.

13.   In a large bowl, combine cooked quinoa, diced vegetables, crumbled feta cheese, chopped fresh parsley, olive oil, lemon juice, salt, and pepper.

14.   Toss gently to combine all ingredients.

15.   Serve as a refreshing and nutritious side dish.

28. Mediterranean Chicken and Vegetable Skillet:

INGREDIENTS:

- Chicken thighs, boneless and skinless
- Cherry tomatoes
- Zucchini
- Red onion
- Garlic
- Kalamata olives
- Olive oil
- Lemon
- Oregano
- Salt and pepper

INSTRUCTIONS:

1.   Season chicken thighs with salt, pepper, and dried oregano.

2.   In a skillet, heat olive oil over medium-high heat.

3.   Brown chicken thighs on both sides until golden.

4.   Add sliced zucchini, halved cherry tomatoes, diced red onion, minced garlic, and Kalamata olives to the skillet.

5.   Squeeze fresh lemon juice over the ingredients.

6.   Continue to cook until the vegetables are tender and the chicken is fully cooked.

7.   Serve hot, garnished with fresh oregano.

29. Mediterranean Couscous Stuffed Bell Peppers:

INGREDIENTS:

- Bell peppers
- Couscous
- Chickpeas
- Feta cheese
- Sun-dried tomatoes
- Fresh parsley
- Olive oil
- Lemon juice
- Garlic
- Oregano
- Salt and pepper

INSTRUCTIONS:

1.   Preheat the oven to 375°F (190°C).

2.   Cut bell peppers in half lengthwise and remove seeds.

3.   Cook couscous according to package instructions.

4.   In a bowl, mix cooked couscous, rinsed chickpeas, crumbled feta cheese, chopped sun-dried tomatoes, chopped fresh parsley, olive oil, lemon juice, minced garlic, oregano, salt, and pepper.

5.   Stuff each bell pepper half with the couscous mixture.

6.   Place the stuffed peppers in a baking dish, cover with foil, and bake for 25-30 minutes or until peppers are tender.

30. *Mediterranean Lemon Garlic Shrimp Pasta:*

INGREDIENTS:

- Shrimp
- Whole wheat pasta
- Cherry tomatoes
- Spinach
- Garlic
- Olive oil
- Lemon zest
- Fresh basil
- Red pepper flakes
- Salt and pepper

INSTRUCTIONS:

1.   Cook whole wheat pasta according to package instructions.

2.   In a skillet, sauté shrimp and minced garlic in olive oil until shrimp are pink and cooked through.

3.   Add halved cherry tomatoes and fresh spinach to the skillet. Cook until spinach wilts.

4.   Toss the cooked pasta into the skillet with the shrimp, tomatoes, and spinach.

5.   Drizzle with olive oil, sprinkle with lemon zest, torn fresh basil, and red pepper flakes.

6.   Toss everything together until well combined.

7.   Serve warm with an additional sprinkle of red pepper flakes if desired.

CONCLUSION

In the final pages of "Wholesome Mediterranean Delights: 30 Inspiring Recipes for a Balanced Lifestyle and Longevity," we find ourselves not just at the conclusion of a culinary adventure but at the gateway to a transformative lifestyle. These 30 recipes, carefully curated from the heart of the Mediterranean, are more than just a collection of dishes; they are a testament to the profound connection between nourishment, joy, and longevity.As we bid farewell to this gastronomic journey, let us carry with us the wisdom ingrained in each recipe—a wisdom born from centuries of tradition and an understanding that food is not merely sustenance but a source of vitality. The Mediterranean diet, celebrated for its health benefits, teaches us that the secret to a balanced life lies in the mindful selection and preparation of ingredients.In our pursuit of longevity, let the echoes of coastal breezes and the laughter around family tables guide us. May the simplicity of olive oil, the vibrancy of herbs, and the richness of seasonal produce become our allies in the quest for a healthier, more wholesome existence. "Wholesome Mediterranean Delights" extends an invitation to not only savor the flavors of the region but to embrace a lifestyle that nurtures the body, uplifts the spirit, and fosters a sense of community. As we close the book, may these recipes linger in our kitchens, inspiring us to create moments of joy, share meals with loved ones, and embark on a journey towards a balanced and fulfilling life, guided by the enduring wisdom of the Mediterranean.